The Mediterranean DIET Cookbook

The best easy-to-prepare recipes.

Christine Hogan

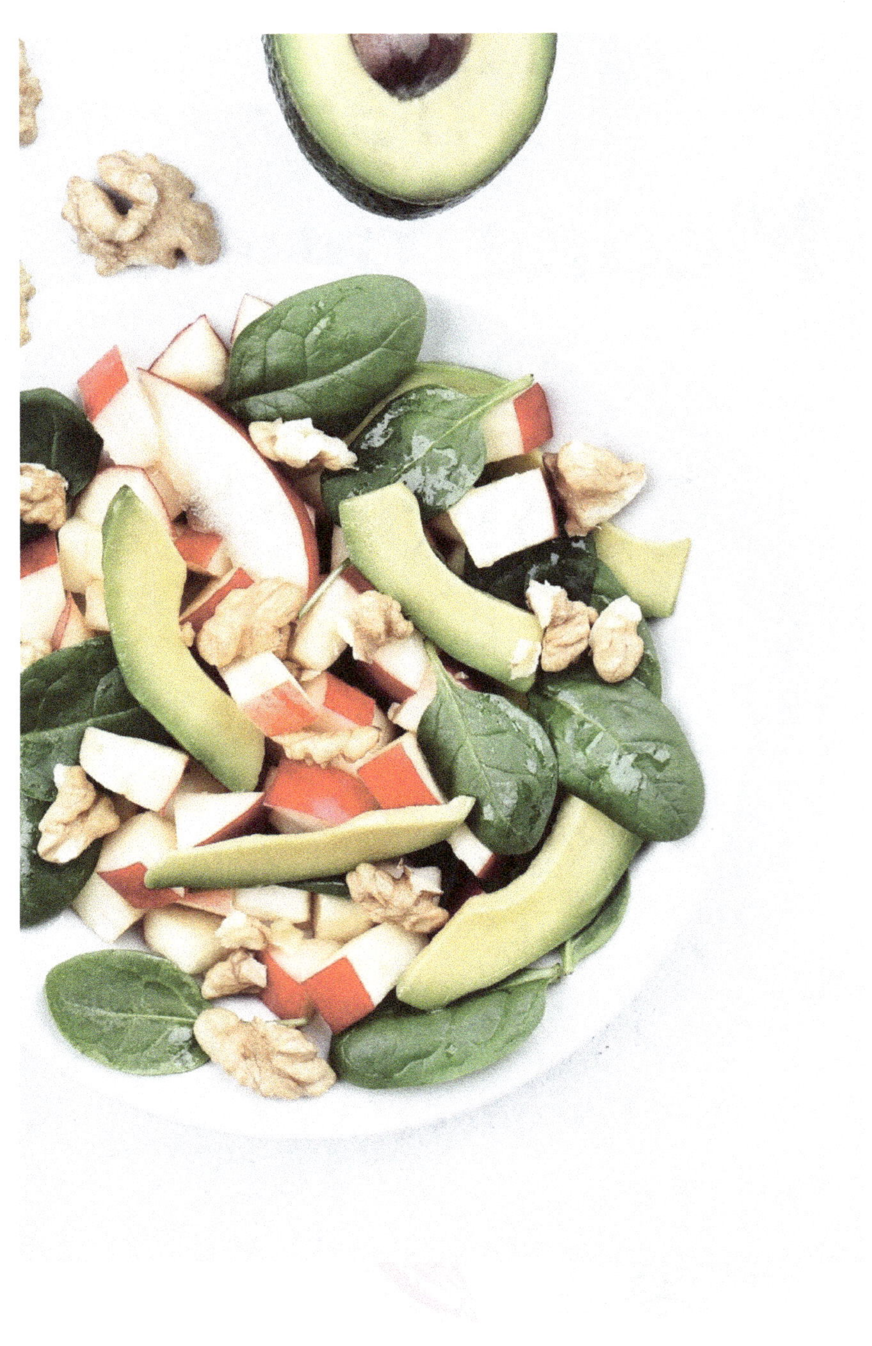

Table of content

MEDITERRANEAN BREAKFAST RECIPE

Creamy Paninis

Total time: 15 minutes

Prep time: 10 minutes

Cook time: 5 minutes

Yield: 4 servings

Ingredients

- 2 tbsp. finely chopped black olives, oil-cured
- ¼ cup chopped fresh basil leaves
- ½ cup mayonnaise dressing with Olive Oil, divided
- 8 slices whole-wheat bread
- 4 slices of bacon
- 1 small zucchini, thinly sliced
- 4 slices provolone cheese
- 7 oz. roasted red peppers, sliced

Directions

- In a small bowl, combine olives, basil, and ¼ cup of mayonnaise; evenly spread the mayonnaise mixture on the bread slices and layer 4 slices with bacon, zucchini, provolone and peppers.
- Top with the remaining bread slices and spread the remaining ¼ cup of mayonnaise on the outside of the sandwiches; cook over medium heat for about 4 minutes, turning once, until cheese is melted and the sandwiches are golden brown.

Breakfast Couscous

Total time: 15 minutes

Prep time: 10 minutes

Cook time: 5 minutes

Yield: 4 servings

Ingredients

- 1 (2-inch) cinnamon stick
- 3 cups 1% low-fat milk
- 1 cup whole-wheat couscous (uncooked)
- 6 tsp. dark brown sugar, divided
- ¼ cup dried currants
- ½ cup chopped apricots (dried)
- ¼ tsp. sea salt
- 4 tsp. melted butter, divided

Directions

- In a saucepan set over medium high heat, combine cinnamon stick and milk; heat for about 3 minutes (do not boil).
- Remove the pan from heat and stir in couscous, 4 teaspoons of sugar, currants, apricots, and sea salt. Let the mixture stand, covered, for at least 15 minutes.
- Discard the cinnamon stick and divide the couscous among four bowls; top each serving with ½ teaspoon of sugar and 1 teaspoon of melted butter. Serve immediately.

Potato and Chickpea Hash

Total time: 15 minutes

Prep time: 10 minutes

Cook time: 5 minutes

Yield: 4 servings

Ingredients

- 4 cups shredded frozen hash brown potatoes
- 1 tbsp. freshly minced ginger
- ½ cup chopped onion
- 2 cups chopped baby spinach
- 1 tbsp. curry powder
- ½ tsp. sea salt
- ¼ cup extra virgin olive oil
- 1 cup chopped zucchini
- 1 (15-ounce) can chickpeas, rinsed
- 4 large eggs

Directions

- In a large bowl, combine the potatoes, ginger, onion, spinach, curry powder, and sea salt.
- In a nonstick skillet set over medium high heat, heat extra virgin olive oil and add the potato mixture.
- Press the mixture into a layer and cook for about 5 minutes, without stirring, or until golden brown and crispy.
- Lower heat to medium low and fold in zucchini and chickpeas, breaking up the mixture until just combined.

- Stir briefly, press the mixture back into a layer, and make four wells.
- Break one egg into each indentation.
- Cook, covered, for about 5 minutes or until eggs are set.

Avocado Toast

Total time: 10 minutes

Prep time: 10 minutes

Cook time: 0 minutes

Yield: 4 servings

Ingredients

- 2 ripe avocados, peeled
- Squeeze of fresh lemon juice, to taste
- 2 tbsp. freshly chopped mint, plus extra to garnish
- Sea salt and black pepper, to taste
- 4 large slices rye bread
- 80 grams soft feta, crumbled

Directions

- In a medium bowl, mash the avocado roughly with a fork; add lemon juice and mint and continue mashing until just combined.
- Season with black pepper and sea salt to taste.
- Grill or toast bread until golden.
- Spread about ¼ of the avocado mixture onto each slice of the toasted bread and top with feta.
- Garnish with extra mint and serve immediately.

Mediterranean Pancakes

Total time: 50 minutes

Prep time: 30 minutes

Cook time: 20 minutes

Yield: 16 Pancakes

Ingredients

- 1 cup old-fashioned oats
- ½ cup all-purpose flour
- 2 tbsp. flax seeds
- 1 tsp. baking soda
- ¼ tsp. sea salt
- 2 tbsp. extra virgin olive oil
- 2 large eggs
- 2 cups nonfat plain Greek yogurt
- 2 tbsp. raw honey
- Fresh fruit, syrup, or other toppings

Directions

- In a blender, combine oats, flour, flax seeds, baking soda, and sea salt; blend for about 30 seconds.
- Add extra virgin olive oil, eggs, yogurt, and honey and continue pulsing until very smooth.
- Let the mixture stand for at least 20 minutes or until thick.
- Set a large nonstick skillet over medium heat and brush with extra virgin olive oil.
- In batches, ladle the batter by quarter-cupfuls into the skillet.

MEDITERRANEAN LUNCH RECIPE

Quinoa Salad with Watermelon and Feta

Serves: 4

Ingredients

- 1 cup Simple Truth Organic™ Quinoa
- 3 tablespoons apple cider vinegar
- 2 tablespoons lemon juice
- 1⁄2 Vidalia onion, finely chopped
- 1⁄2 cup Simple Truth Organic™ Unfiltered Extra Virgin Olive Oil
- Coarse salt, to taste
- Freshly ground pepper, to taste
- 3⁄4 cup crumbled feta cheese
- 1⁄2 seedless watermelon, (about 1½ cups) diced
- 3 tablespoons Italian parsley, minced

Directions

- Cook quinoa according to package directions. Rinse with cold water and drain.
- To make dressing: in a small bowl or jar, combine vinegar, lemon juice and onion. Mix well and add in olive oil and whisk well to emulsify dressing. Season with salt and pepper to taste.
- In a medium bowl, combine the cooked quinoa with feta, watermelon, parsley and dressing. Add salt and pepper to taste. Serve chilled or at room temperature.

Mediterranean Orzo

Serves: 8

Ingredients

- 14 ounces orzo pasta
- 1 tablespoon Simple Extra Virgin Olive Oil
- 1 jar (8.5 oz.) sun-dried tomatoes in oil, julienne cut
- 8 green onions, chopped
- 4 ounces feta cheese
- 1⁄4 cup provolone cheese, shredded
- 1 jar (16 oz.) Italian dressing

Directions

- Cook pasta in a large saucepan of boiling water with 1 tablespoon olive oil. Cook until done but still firm to bite. Drain and allow to cool.
- In a large bowl, combine pasta, sun-dried tomatoes, green onions, feta cheese and provolone. Pour dressing over top. Stir to combine.

Meyer Lemon Quinoa Skillet

Ingredients

- 2 teaspoons olive oil
- 1⁄2 cup onion, chopped
- 1 teaspoon minced garlic
- 1 can (15.5 oz.) cannellini beans, drained and rinsed
- 1 can (14 oz.) quartered artichoke hearts, drained and roughly chopped
- 2 packages (10 oz.) Simple Truth Organic White Quinoa with Olive Oil & Sea Salt
- 1⁄4 cup water
- 2 Meyer lemons, zested and juiced
- 1⁄2 teaspoon salt
- 1⁄4 teaspoon ground black pepper
- 2 tablespoons flat leaf parsley, chopped
- 4 ounces crumbled feta cheese

Directions

- In medium non-stick skillet over medium heat, heat oil. Cook onion and garlic 2 to 3 minutes, until translucent.
- Stir in beans, artichokes, quinoa and water. Cook 4 to 6 minutes until hot.
- Stir in lemon juice, salt, pepper and parsley. Adjust seasoning to taste.
- Serve topped with feta cheese and lemon zest.

Creamy Corn, Squash and Cilantro

Serves: 8

Ingredients

- 4 cloves garlic, minced and divided
- 1/4 cup cilantro, minced
- 1/2 cup mayonnaise
- 2 tablespoons sour cream
- 1/4 teaspoon salt
- 1 bag (10 oz.) Simple Truth Organic™ Whole Kernel Cut Corn
- 3 tablespoons Olive oil
- 1 zucchini, washed and chopped
- 1 yellow squash, washed and chopped
- 1/2 cup queso fresco, crumbled

Directions

- Heat grill to 250°F.
- To make aioli, mix 2 garlic cloves, mayonnaise, sour cream and salt in a small bowl.
- Cook corn in microwave as directed on the package.
- Heat oil in cast iron skillet and place on the grill. Add 2 minced garlic cloves and cook, uncovered, for 30 seconds. Add zucchini and yellow squash and cook for 3-5 minutes, turning occasionally, until vegetables are crisp-tender. Add corn and cook until vegetables are cooked through.
- Serve vegetables with aioli and queso fresco on the side.

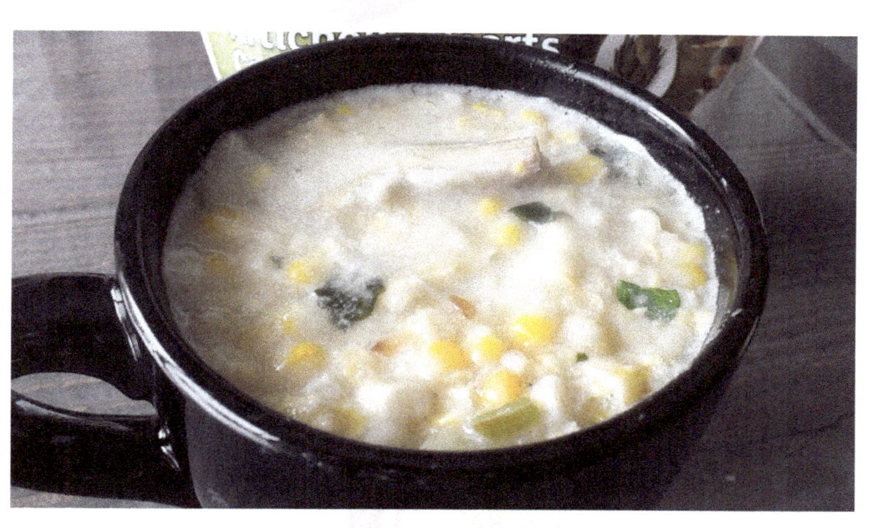

Mediterranean Turkey and Rice Skillet

Serves: 5

Ingredients

- 1 tablespoon olive oil
- 1 pound ground turkey
- 1 small onion, chopped
- 2 teaspoons minced garlic
- 1 teaspoon salt
- 1/2 teaspoon ground black pepper
- 1/2 teaspoon dried oregano
- 1/2 cup Private Selection Sun-Dried Tomatoes, drained and roughly chopped
- 1 cup long grain white rice
- 2 cups chicken broth
- 5 ounces baby spinach
- 1 lemon, zested and juiced
- 1/2 cup feta cheese crumbles

Directions

- In large skillet over medium-high heat, heat oil. Cook ground turkey, onion, garlic, salt, pepper and oregano until meat is browned and onion is translucent.
- Mix in sun-dried tomatoes, rice and chicken broth. Bring to boil. Cover and reduce heat to low. Cook 15 minutes, until rice is tender.
- Stir in spinach, lemon juice and zest. Continue cooking until spinach is wilted.

- Serve topped with feta cheese.

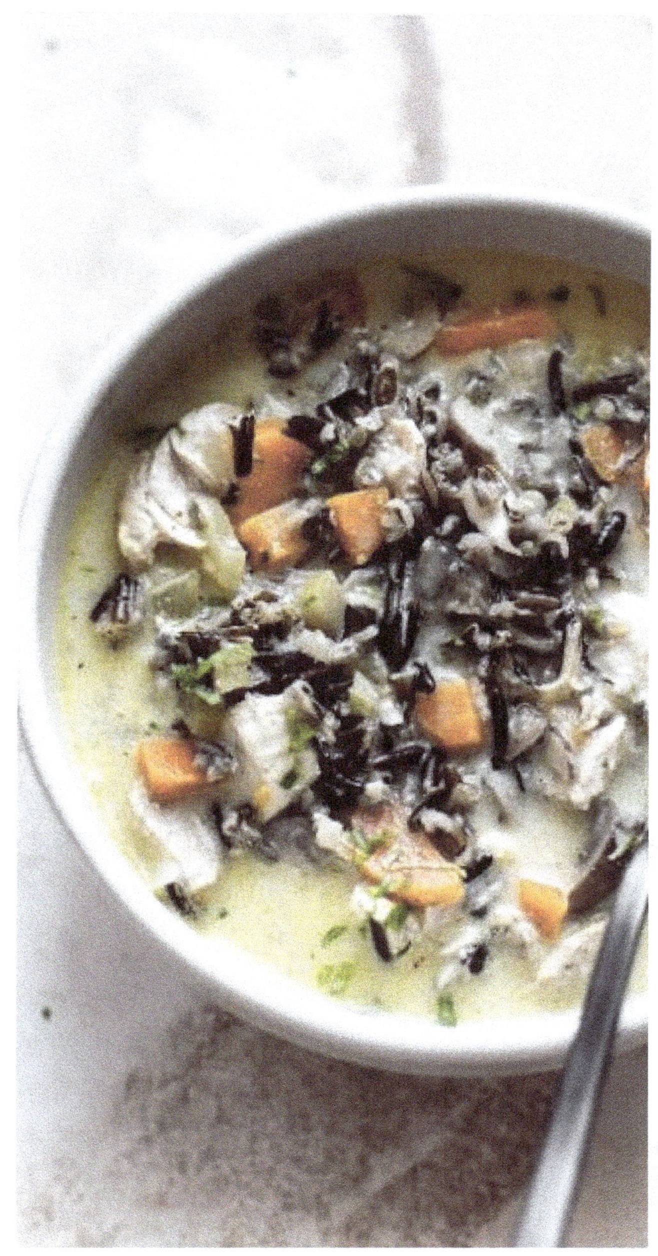

Mediterranean Quinoa Stuffed Peppers

Ingredients

- 2 large red bell peppers
- 1 cup cooked quinoa
- 1 cup low sodium cooked chickpeas
- 1 cup cherry tomatoes, quartered
- 2 tablespoons pine nuts
- 2 tablespoons sliced black olives
- 1 clove garlic
- 1 teaspoon red wine vinegar
- 1 teaspoon dried oregano
- Chopped parsley, for serving (optional)

Preparation

- Heat oven to 350F.
- Cut bell peppers vertically down the center in half and remove stems and seeds. Place peppers on a baking sheet lined with parchment or a silicone baking mat.
- In a mixing bowl, combine remaining ingredients. Scoop mixture into pepper halves.
- Bake for 20 to 25 minutes, or until peppers are soft but still hold their shape. Remove from oven and sprinkle with parsley before serving (optional).

Japanese Onigiri Rice Triangles Recipe

Ingredients

- 1½ cups uncooked short grain white rice
- 1 2/3 cups water
- ½ teaspoon salt
- ½ ounce dried sliced seaweed, finely chopped (2 tablespoons)
- 1 tablespoon sesame seeds
- 4 ounces cooked, smoked, or canned salmon
- 1 sheet nori

Preparation

- Measure the rice in a medium saucepan. Rinse, stir, and drain it several times. Cover it with plenty of water and allow it to soak for about 40 minutes or until the rice is an opaque white color. Thoroughly drain the rice in a mesh strainer.
- Return the drained rice to the saucepan. Add water and salt; cover the pot. Bring it to a boil over high heat, then reduce heat to maintain a simmer. Cook the rice for 20 minutes, then remove it from the heat. Leave the pot covered and allow the rice to steam for another 10 minutes to finish the cooking process.
- Sprinkle in the seaweed and sesame seeds. Stir to combine.
- When the rice mixture is cool enough to handle, moisten both hands. Spread about ½ cup of the rice out on the palm

of one hand. Place 1 tablespoon of salmon in the center, and form the rice mixture into a ball around it. Press firmly to stick the rice together. Form it into the traditional triangle shape, flat on both sides, with rounded corners.

- Using scissors, cut the sheet of nori into strips, 1 x 2 ½-inches each; wrap a strip of nori around one edge of the triangle. Cover or wrap tightly until serving.

MEDITERRANEAN SALAD RECIPES

Grilled Tofu with Mediterranean Salad

Total time: 45 minutes

Prep time: 30 minutes

Cook time: 15 minutes

Yield: 4 servings

Ingredients

- 1 tbsp. extra virgin olive oil
- ¼ cup lemon juice
- 2 tsp. dried oregano
- 3 cloves garlic, minced
- ½ tsp. sea salt
- Freshly ground pepper
- 14 ounces water-packed extra-firm tofu
- Mediterranean Chopped Salad
- 2 tbsp. extra virgin olive oil
- ¼ cup coarsely chopped Kalamata olives
- ¼ cup chopped scallions
- 1 cup diced seedless cucumber
- 2 medium tomatoes, diced
- ¼ cup chopped fresh parsley
- 1 tbsp. white-wine vinegar
- Freshly ground pepper
- ¼ tsp. sea salt

Directions

- Preheat your grill.

- In a small bowl, combine extra virgin olive oil, lemon juice, oregano, garlic, sea salt and black pepper; reserve two tablespoons of the mixture for basting.
- Drain tofu and rinse; pat dry with paper towels. Cut tofu crosswise into 8 ½-inch thick slices and put in a glass dish.
- Add the lemon juice marinade and turn tofu to coat well.
- Marinate in the fridge for at least 30 minutes.
- In the meantime, prepare the salad.
- In a medium bowl, combine all the salad ingredients; toss gently to mix well.
- Set aside.
- Brush the grill rack with oil. Drain the marinated tofu and discard the marinade.
- Grill tofu over medium heat, for about 4 minutes per side, basting frequently with the remaining lemon juice marinade.
- Serve grilled tofu warm, topped with the salad.

Mediterranean Barley Salad

Total time: 1 hour 45 minutes

Prep time: 15 minutes

Cook time: 30 minutes

Chilling time: 1 hour

Yield: 6 servings

Ingredients

- 2 ½ cups water
- 1 cup barley
- 4 tbsp. extra virgin olive oil, divided
- 2 cloves garlic
- 7 sun-dried tomatoes
- 1 tbsp. balsamic vinegar
- ½ cup chopped black olives
- ½ cup finely chopped cilantro

Directions

- Mix water and barley in a saucepan; bring the mixture to a rolling boil over high heat.
- Lower heat to medium-low and simmer, covered, for about 30 minutes or until tender, but still a bit firm in the center.
- Drain and transfer to a large bowl; let the cooked barley cool to room temperature.
- In a blender, puree 2 tablespoons of extra virgin olive oil, garlic, sun-dried tomatoes, and balsamic vinegar until very smooth; pour over barley and fold in the remaining olive oil, olives, and cilantro.

- Refrigerate, covered, until chilled.
- Stir to mix well before serving.

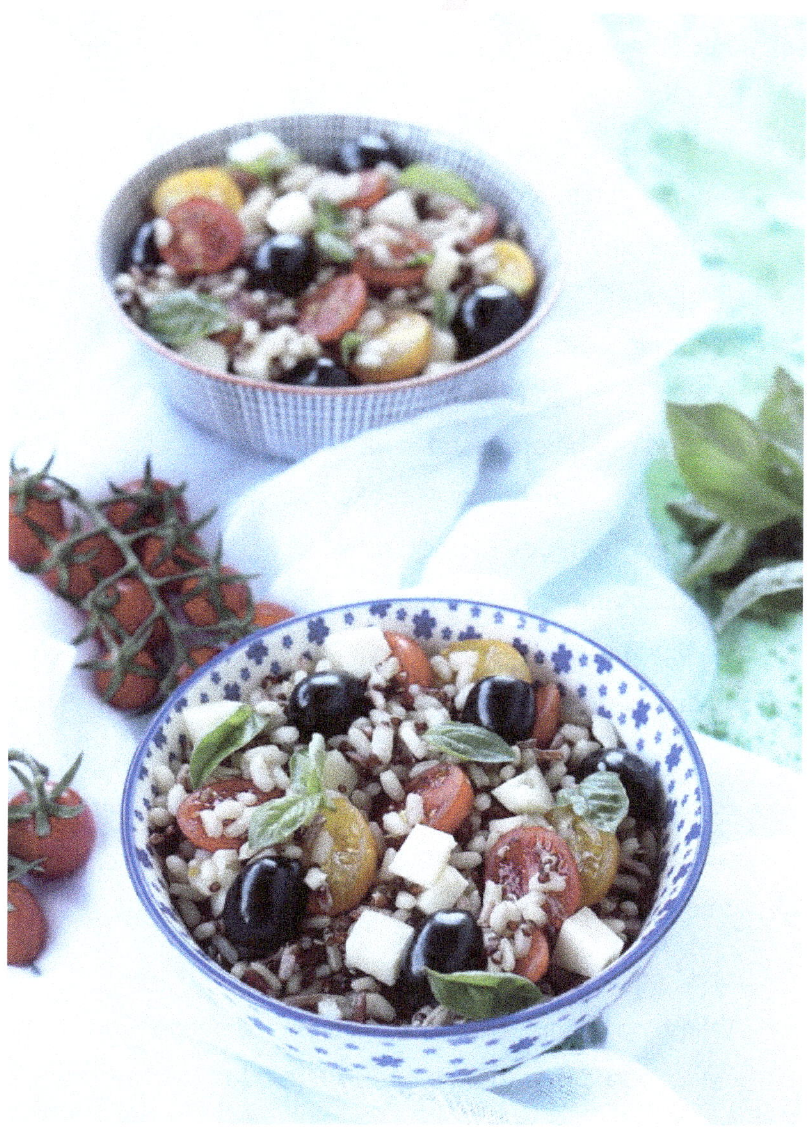

Mediterranean Quinoa Salad

Total time: 35 minutes

Prep time: 15 minutes

Cook time: 20 minutes

Yield: 4 servings

Ingredients

- 1 clove garlic, smashed
- 2 cups water
- 2 cubes chicken bouillon
- 1 cup uncooked quinoa
- ½ cup chopped Kalamata olives
- 1 large red onion, diced
- 2 large chicken breasts (cooked), diced
- 1 large green bell pepper, diced
- ½ cup crumbled feta cheese
- ¼ cup chopped fresh chives
- ¼ cup chopped fresh parsley
- ½ tsp. sea salt
- ¼ cup extra virgin olive oil
- 1 tbsp. balsamic vinegar
- ⅔ cup fresh lemon juice

Directions

- Combine garlic clove, water, and bouillon cubes in a saucepan; bring the mixture to a gentle boil over medium-low heat.

- Stir in quinoa and simmer, covered, for about 20 minutes or until the water has been absorbed and quinoa is tender.
- Discard garlic clove and transfer the cooked quinoa to a large bowl.
- Stir in olives, onion, chicken, bell pepper, feta cheese, chives, parsley, sea salt, extra virgin olive oil, balsamic vinegar, and lemon juice.
- Serve warm or chilled.

MEDITERRANEAN POULTRY RECIPES

Chicken Bruschetta

Total time: 30 minutes

Prep time: 10 minutes

Cook time: 20 minutes

Yield: 4 servings

Ingredients

- 5ml olive oil, divided
- 1 boneless, skinless chicken breast
- 80g cherry tomatoes
- 5ml balsamic vinegar
- 10g fresh basil leaves
- 1 small cloves garlic, minced
- 1 small onions, chopped

Directions

- Add half of the oil to the skillet and cook chicken over medium heat.
- In the meantime, cut basil leaves into slivers and prepare the vegetables.
- Heat the remaining oil and sauté garlic and onion for about 3 minutes.
- Stir in basil and tomatoes for about 5 minutes.
- Stir in vinegar.
- Cook until heated through and serve the chicken topped with onion and tomato mixture.

Coconut Chicken

Total time: 30 minutes

Prep time: 20 minutes

Cook time: 10 minutes

Yield: 4 servings

Ingredients

- 20g coconut, shredded
- 30g almond flour
- 1 tsp. sea salt
- 1 small egg
- 100g chicken breast, boneless, skinless
- 7.5 ml coconut oil

Directions

- In a bowl, combine shredded coconut, almond flour and sea salt.
- In a separate bowl, beat the egg; dip the chicken in the egg and roll in the flour mixture until well coated.
- Add coconut oil to a pan set over medium heat and fry the chicken until the crust begins to brown.
- Transfer the chicken to the oven and bake at 350°F for about 10 minutes.

Turkey Burgers

Total time: 25 minutes

Prep time: 15 minutes

Cook time: 10 minutes

Yield: 4 servings

Ingredients

- 1 large egg white
- 1 cup red onion, chopped
- ¾ cup fresh mint, chopped
- ½ cup dried bread crumbs
- 1 tsp. dill, dried
- ⅓ cup feta cheese, crumbled
- ¾ kg turkey, ground
- Cooking spray
- 4 hamburger buns, split
- 1 red bell pepper, roasted and cut in strips
- 2 tbsp. fresh lime juice

Directions

- Lightly beat the egg white in a bowl and add onion, mint, breadcrumbs, dill, cheese, turkey and lime juice, mix well then divide the turkey mixture into four equal burger patties.
- Spray a large nonstick skillet with cooking spray and heat on medium-high setting.
- Carefully place the patties in the skillet and cook for 8 minutes on each side or according to preference.

- Once cooked, place the burgers on the sliced buns and top with pepper strips.

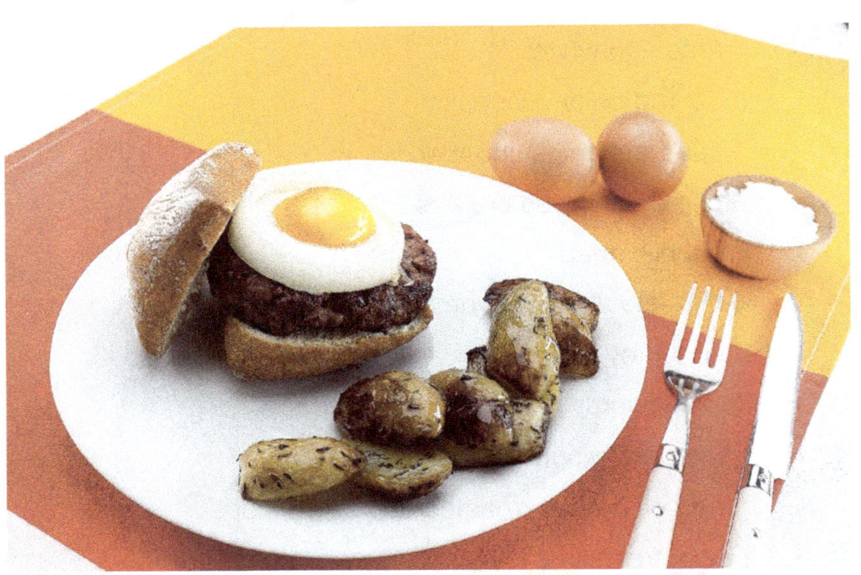

Chicken with Greek Salad

Total time: 25 minutes

Prep time: 25 minutes

Cook time: 0 minutes

Yield: 4 servings

Ingredients

- 2 tbsp. extra virgin olive oil
- ⅓ cup red-wine vinegar
- 1 tsp. garlic powder
- 1 tbsp. chopped fresh dill
- ¼ tsp. sea salt
- ¼ tsp. freshly ground pepper
- 2 ½ cups chopped cooked chicken
- 6 cups chopped romaine lettuce
- 1 cucumber, peeled, seeded and chopped
- 2 medium tomatoes, chopped
- ½ cup crumbled feta cheese
- ½ cup sliced ripe black olives
- ½ cup finely chopped red onion

Directions

- In a large bowl, whisk together extra virgin olive oil, vinegar, garlic powder, dill, sea salt and pepper.
- Add chicken, lettuce, cucumber, tomatoes, feta, and olives and toss to combine well. Enjoy!

MEDITERRANEAN SEAFOOD RECIPES

Salmon and Vegetable Kedgeree

Total time: 30 minutes

Prep time: 10 minutes

Cook time: 20 minutes

Ingredients

- 60ml basmati rice
- 7.5ml extra virgin olive oil
- 2g curry powder
- 100g skinless hot-smoked salmon portions, flaked
- 100g vegetable mix
- Sea salt and pepper, to taste
- 1 green onion, thinly sliced

Directions

- In a saucepan of boiling salted water, add rice, turn heat to low and cook, covered, until just tender, for about 12 minutes.
- Add extra virgin olive oil to a pan set over medium heat and cook the onion, stirring until tender, for about 3 minutes.
- Stir in curry powder and continue cooking until fragrant, for about 1 minute.
- Stir in rice until well combined and then add salmon, vegetables, salt and pepper.
- Continue cooking until heated through, for about 3 minutes.
- Serve.

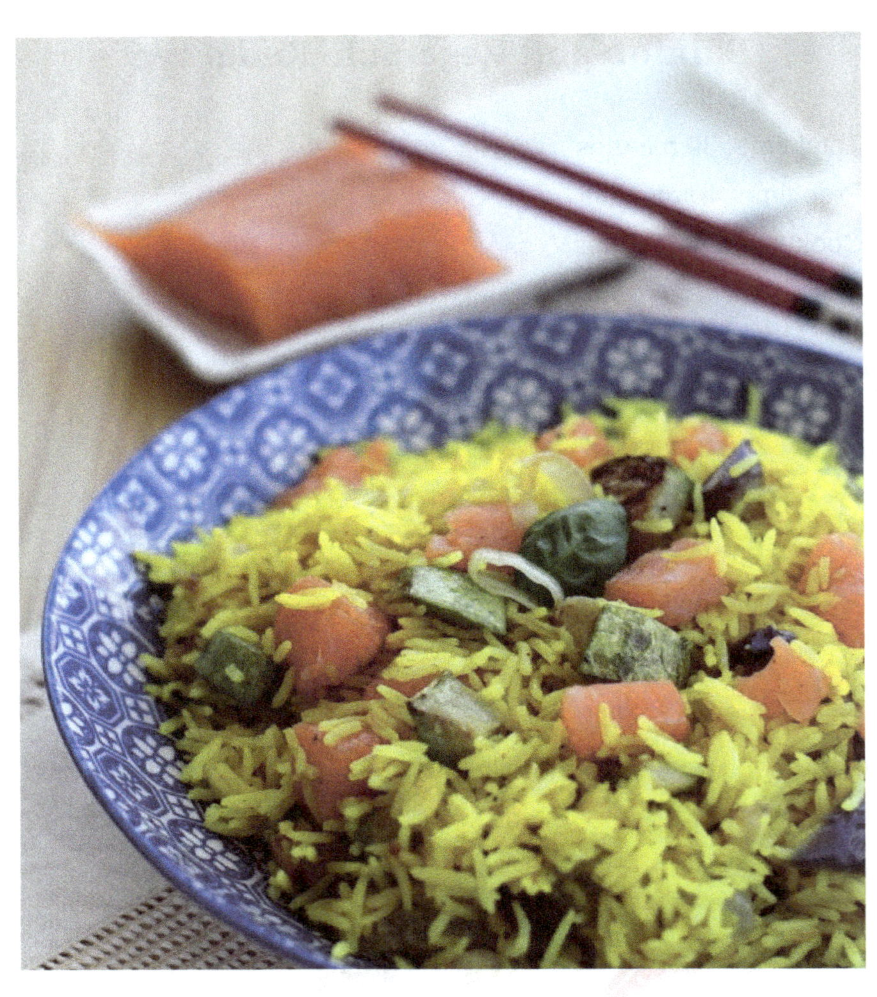

Grilled Sardines with Wilted Arugula

Total time: 25 minutes

Prep time: 15 minutes

Cook time: 10 minutes

Servings: 4

Ingredients

- 2 large bunches baby arugula, trimmed
- 16 fresh sardines, innards and gills removed
- 2 tsp. extra virgin olive oil
- Sea salt
- Freshly ground black pepper
- Lemon wedges, for garnish

Directions

- Prepare your outdoor grill or a stove-top griddle.
- Rinse arugula under running water; shake off excess water and arrange them on a platter; set aside.
- Rinse sardines in water and rub to remove scales; wipe them dry and combine with extra virgin olive oil in a large bowl.
- Toss to coat.
- Place the sardines over the grill and grill for about 3 minutes per side or until golden brown and crispy.
- Season with sea salt and pepper and immediately transfer to the platter lined with arugula.
- Serve right away garnished with lemon wedges.

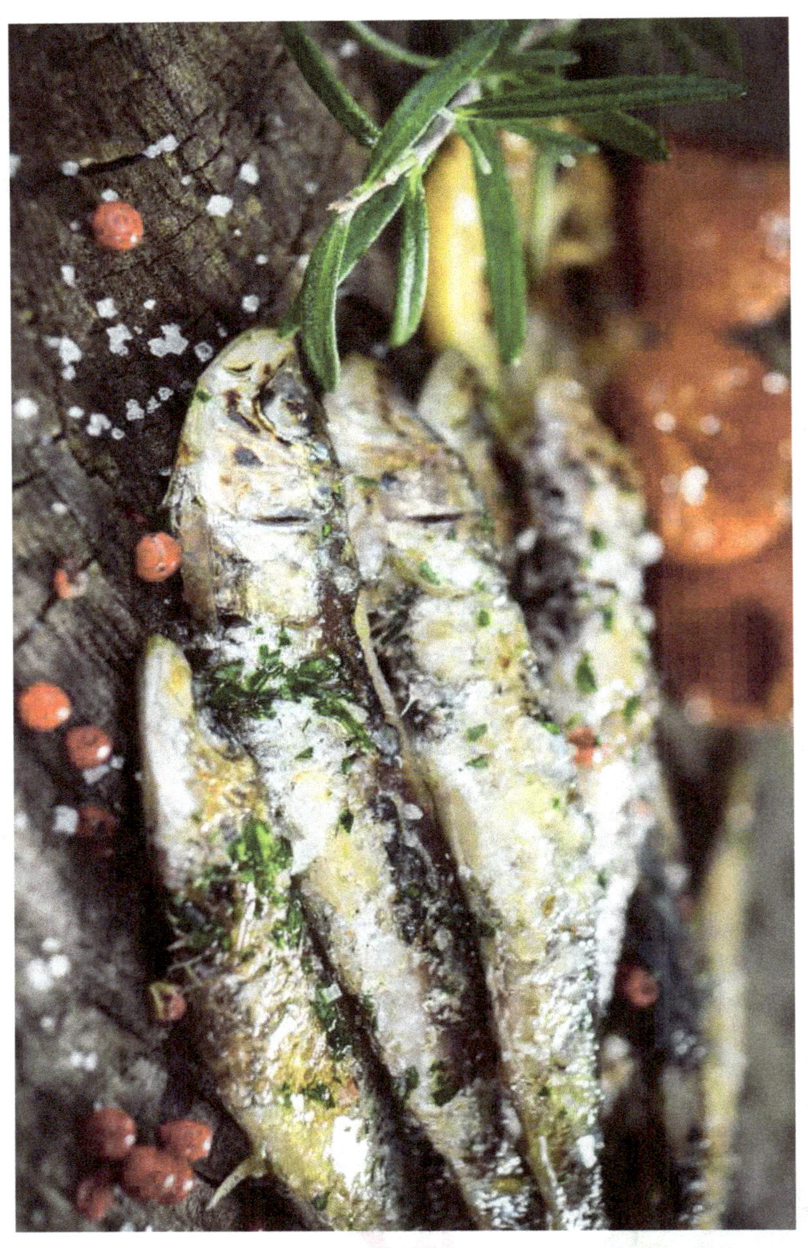

Curry Salmon with Napa Slaw

Total time: 1 hour

Prep time: 15 minutes

Cook time: 45 minutes

Yield: 4 servings

Ingredients

- 1 cup brown basmati rice
- A pinch of coarse salt
- A pinch of ground black pepper
- 1 pound (½ head) Napa cabbage, sliced crosswise
- 2 tbsp. extra virgin olive oil
- ¼ cup freshly squeezed lime juice
- ½ cup fresh mint leaves
- 1 pound carrots, coarsely grated
- 4 (6 ounces each) salmon filets
- 2 tsp. curry powder
- Lime wedges for serving

Directions

- Bring two cups of water to a gentle boil in a large saucepan set over medium-low heat; add rice and season with sea salt and pepper; turn heat to low and cook, covered, for about 35 minutes.
- In the meantime, combine Napa cabbage, extra virgin olive oil, lime juice, mint, carrots, salt and black pepper in a large bowl; toss until well combined.
- Set broiler rack 4 inches from heat and preheat it.

- Place salmon in a baking sheet lined with foil and rub it with curry, salt and pepper.
- Broil the fish for about 8 minutes or until just cooked through.
- Serve the cooked rice alongside green salad and grilled salmon.

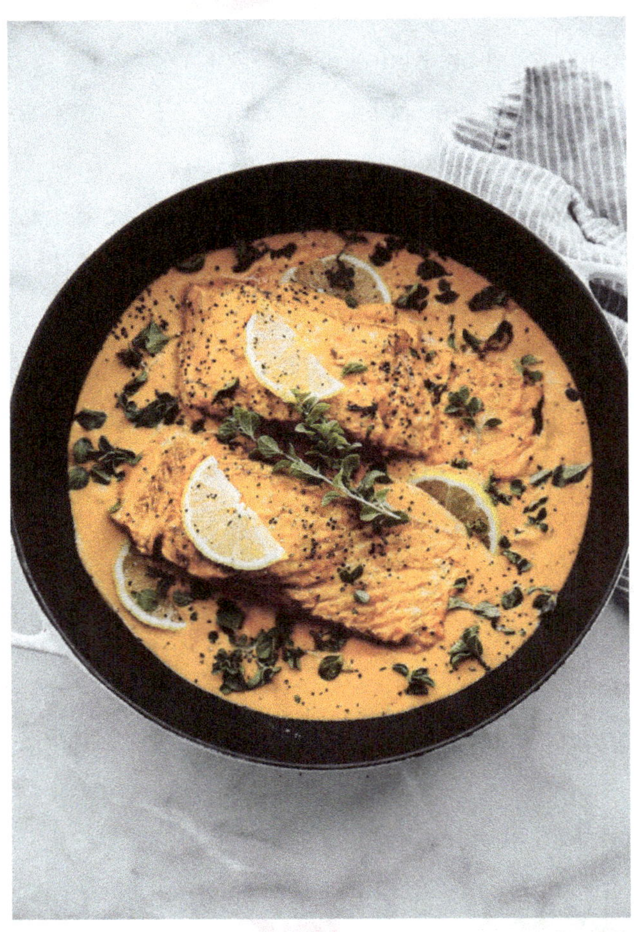

Shrimp and Pasta

Total time: 20 minutes

Prep time: 15 minutes

Cook time: 5 minutes

Yield: 4 servings

Ingredients

- 2 tsp. extra virgin olive oil
- 2 garlic cloves, minced
- 1 pound shrimp, peeled, deveined
- 2 cups chopped plum tomato
- ¼ cup thinly sliced fresh basil
- 2 tbsp. capers, drained
- ⅓ cup chopped pitted Kalamata olives
- ¼ tsp. freshly ground black pepper
- 4 cups hot cooked angel hair pasta
- ¼ cup crumbled feta cheese
- Cooking spray

Directions

- In a large nonstick skillet set over medium high heat, heat extra virgin olive oil; add garlic and sauté for about 30 seconds.
- Add shrimp and sauté for 1 minute more.
- Stir in tomato and basil and lower heat to medium low; simmer for about 3 minutes or until the tomato is tender.
- Stir in capers, Kalamata olives and black pepper.

- In a large bowl, combine pasta and shrimp mixture; toss to mix and top with cheese.
- Serve immediately.

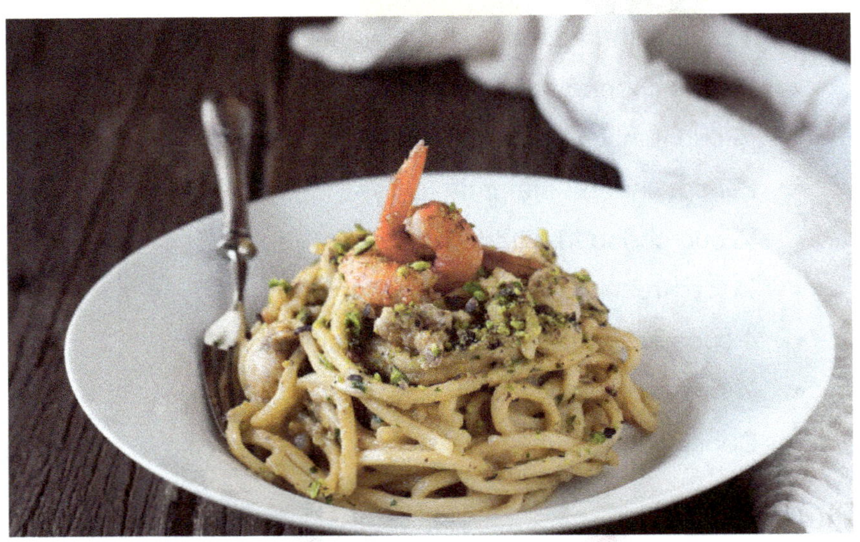

MEDITERRANEAN MEAT, BEEF AND PORK RECIPES

Liver with Apple and Onion

Total time: 35 minutes

Prep time: 10 minutes

Cook time: 25 minutes

Yield: 2 servings

Ingredients

- Extra virgin olive oil spray
- ½ lb. onion
- 2 Granny Smith apples
- 1 cup water
- 1 tbsp. fresh lemon juice
- 1 tbsp. white wine vinegar
- 1 tsp. brown sugar
- 1 tbsp. fresh rosemary, plus sprigs for garnish
- 2 tbsp. dried currants
- 2 tsp. unsalted butter
- 8 ounces calves' liver
- ¼ cup white wine
- ¼ tsp. sea salt
- olive oil spray

Directions

- Preheat your oven to 200ºF.
- Spray skillet with extra virgin olive oil spray and set over medium heat; add onions and sauté for about 4 minutes or until translucent.

- Add apples and cook for about 5 minutes or until they start to brown.
- Stir in water, lemon juice, vinegar and sugar and cook until apples are tender.
- Stir in rosemary and currants, cook, stirring for about 2 minutes and divide between two plates; keep warm in the oven.
- Melt butter in the same pan until frothing.
- Stir in liver and sauté for about 10 minutes or until browned on the outside.
- Divide the liver between the two plates of apple-onion mixture.
- Add white wine to the hot pan to deglaze; cook until the liquid is reduced by half and pour equal amounts over each serving.
- Serve garnished with fresh rosemary.

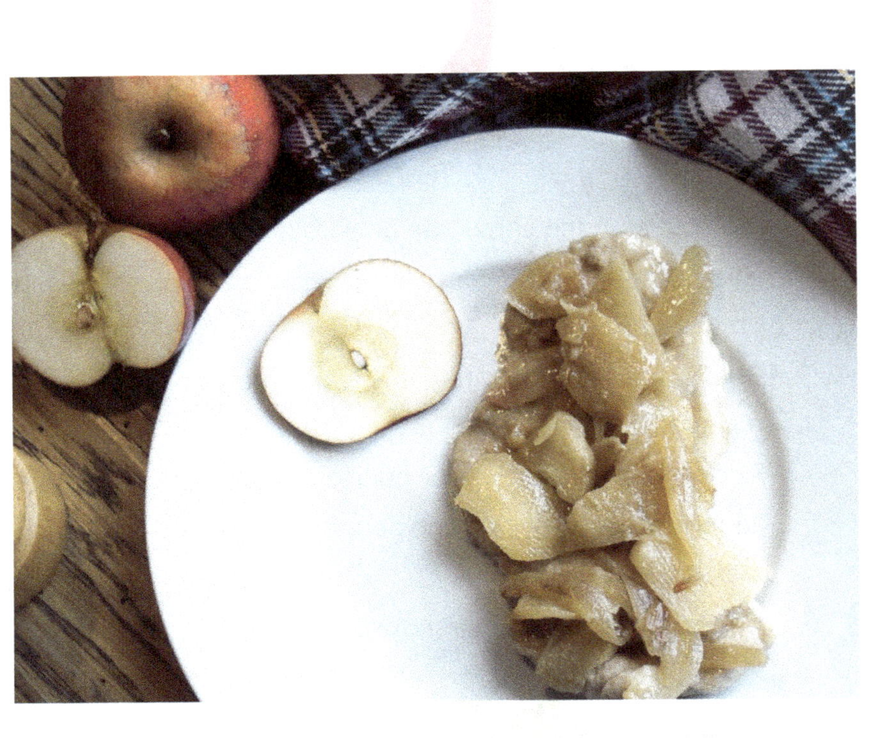

Lamb Chops

Total time: 25 minutes

Prep time: 10 minutes

Cook time: 10 minutes

Standing time: 5 minutes

Yield: 4 servings

Ingredients

- 1 tbsp. dried oregano
- 1 tbsp. garlic, minced
- ¼ tsp. black pepper, freshly ground
- ½ tsp. sea salt
- 2 tbsp. lemon juice, fresh
- 8 lamb loin chops, fat trimmed off
- Cooking spray

Directions

- Preheat your broiler.
- In a small bowl, combine all the spices, herbs and lemon juice and rub this mixture on both sides of the lamb chops.
- Spray the broiler pan with the cooking spray and broil the lamb chops for 4 minutes on each side or depending on how done you want your chops. Cover the cooked lamb chops in foil and let them rest for 5 minutes and you are ready to serve.

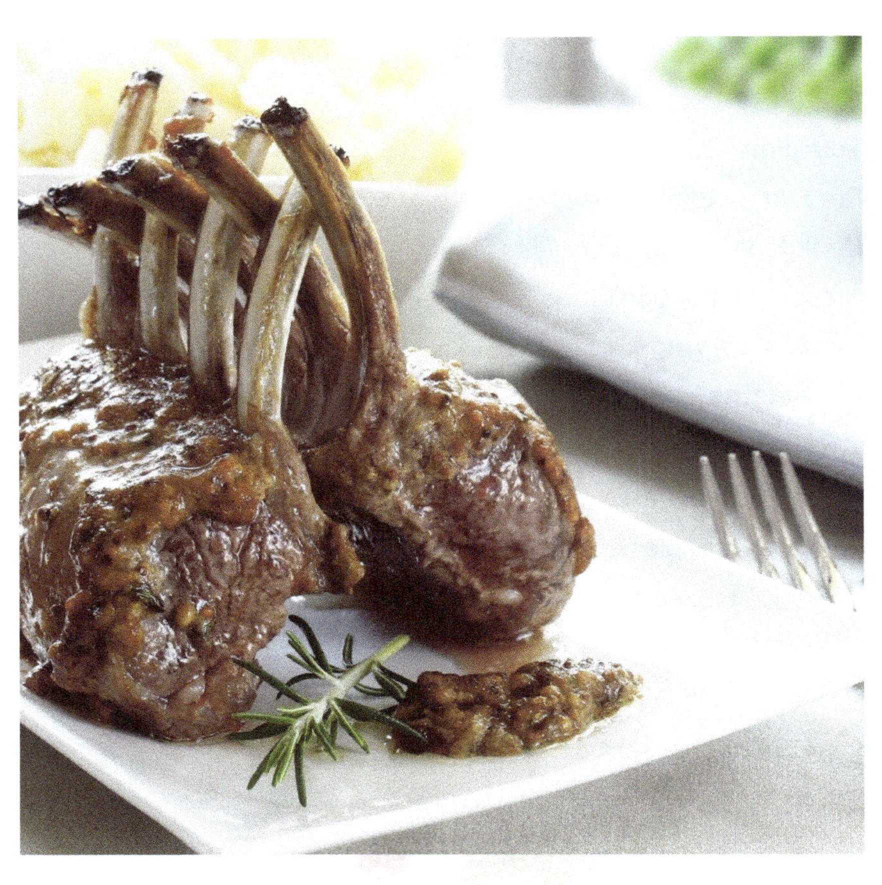

Sage Seared Calf's Liver

Total time: 30 minutes

Prep time: 20 minutes

Cook time: 10 minutes

Yield: 4 servings

Ingredients

- 2 tsp. extra virgin olive oil
- 1 clove garlic, minced
- 8 ounces calves' liver, cut into small strips
- 1 tbsp. flat leaf parsley
- 1 tbsp. fresh sage
- 1 tsp. balsamic vinegar
- 2 tbsp. red wine
- 2 tsp. unsalted butter
- 1 tsp. fresh lemon juice
- ¼ tsp. sea salt
- Black pepper

Directions

- Heat extra virgin olive oil in a nonstick skillet set over medium heat; stir in minced garlic and sauté for about 3 minutes or until translucent and fragrant.
- Add strips of liver, parsley and sage and cook for about 5 minutes or until the meat is seared on outside.
- Transfer the liver to a warm plate and quickly deglaze the pan with vinegar, red wine, butter, and lemon juice for about 30 seconds.

- Pour the sauce over the meat and serve right away.

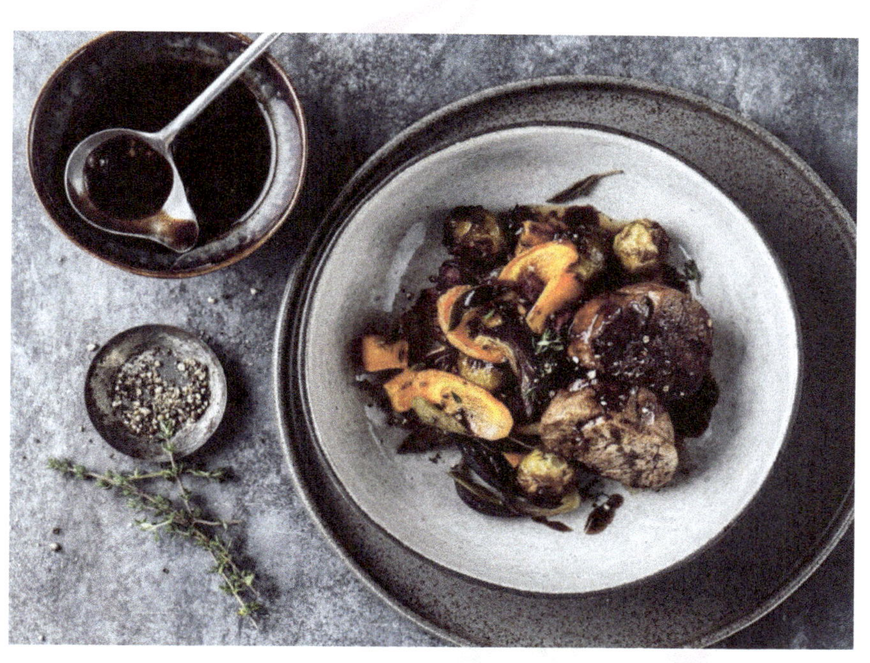

Seasoned Lamb Burgers

Total time: 30 minutes

Prep time: 20 minutes

Cook time: 10 minutes

Yield: 4 servings

Ingredients

- 1 ½ pounds ground lamb
- 1 tsp. ground cumin
- ½ tsp. ground cinnamon
- 1 tsp. ground ginger
- ¼ cup extra virgin olive oil, divided
- 1 tsp. black pepper, freshly ground; divided
- ¼ cup fresh cilantro
- 2 tbsp. fresh oregano
- 1 small clove garlic, pressed
- ¾ tsp. red pepper flakes, crushed
- ¼ cup fresh flat leaf parsley
- 1 tbsp. sherry vinegar
- 2 pitas, warmed and halved
- Sliced tomato
- 1 8 oz of package plain Greek yogurt

Directions

- Prepare a charcoal or gas grill fire.
- Mix the ground lamb with cumin, cinnamon, ginger, 1 tablespoon extra virgin olive oil and ½ teaspoon black pepper.

- Mix well and divide this into four burgers.

- Spray the grill with some olive oil and grill the burgers for 5 minutes on each side.

- Combine the rest of the olive oil, cilantro, oregano, garlic, red pepper flakes, parsley and vinegar in a food processor until it forms a thick paste. Serve each burger in pita bread on a plate with sliced tomato, the processed sauce and a serving of yogurt.

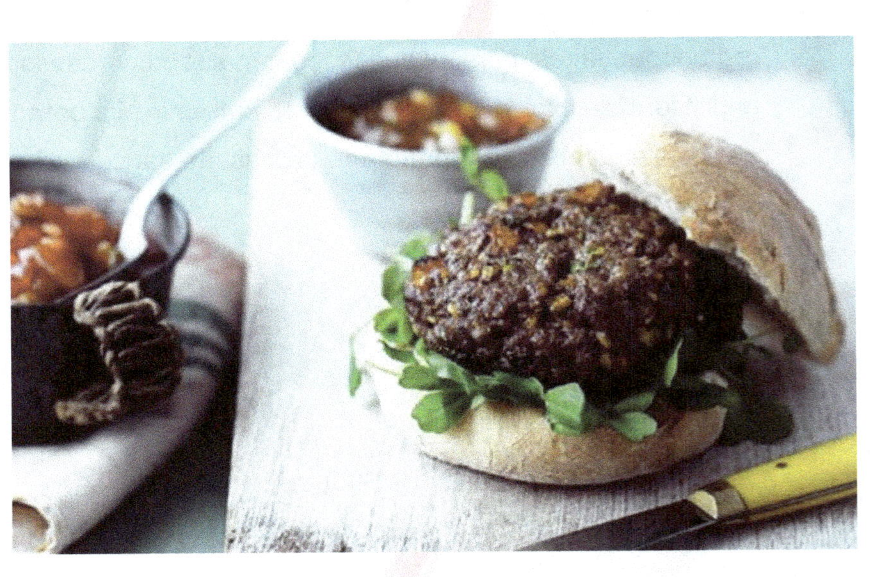

VEGETARIAN AND LEGUMES MEDITERRANEAN RECIPES

Stewed Artichokes with Beans

Total time: 40 minutes

Prep time: 15 minutes

Cook time: 25 minutes

Yield: 4 servings

Ingredients

- 1 ½ pounds fava beans, shelled
- 3 tbsp. freshly squeezed lemon juice
- 4 cups water
- 24 baby artichokes
- 1 lemon half, to rub artichokes
- 2 tsp. extra virgin olive oil
- 4 sprigs fresh flat-leaf parsley
- 4 sprigs fresh thyme
- 1/4 tsp. crushed red-pepper flakes
- 1/4 tsp. freshly ground black pepper
- 1 tsp. sea salt
- 3 peeled and lightly crushed cloves garlic
- 1 lemon half, to rub artichokes

Directions

- Fill a large bowl with water and ice; set aside.
- Add water to a medium pot and bring to a rolling boil over high heat.
- Add fava beans and blanch for about 30 seconds.
- Remove the beans from hot water and add to a bowl with ice bath; let soak for about 5 minutes or until cold.

- Peel the skin from the fava beans and set aside.

- In a large bowl, combine lemon juice with 4 cups of water; set aside.

- Remove the tough outer leaves from the artichokes and cut off the tips.

- Trim each stem and peel; rub with the lemon half and place in the lemon-water mixture.

- Add extra virgin olive oil to a saucepan set over medium heat; heat until hot but not smoky.

- Add garlic, red pepper flakes, sea salt and black pepper; cook, stirring, for about 2 minutes or until the shallot is lightly browned.

- Stir in the artichokes, parsley, thyme, and 1 cup of lemon-water mixture; bring the mixture to a gentle simmer.

- Lower heat to medium low and continue simmering, covered, for about 14 minutes or until the artichokes are tender.

- Add the fava beans and continue cooking for 3 minutes more or until the beans are tender. Serve immediately.

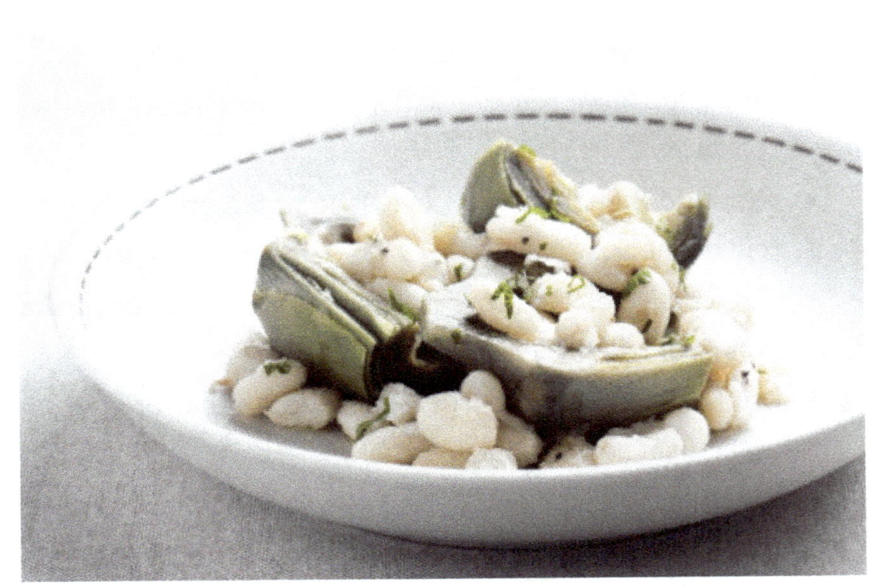

Mediterranean Pasta with Olives, Tomatoes and Artichokes

Total time: 35 minutes

Prep time: 15 minutes

Cook time: 20 minutes

Yield: 4 servings

Ingredients

- 12 ounces whole-wheat spaghetti
- 2 tbsp. extra virgin olive oil, divided
- 2 garlic cloves, sliced
- ½ medium onion, thinly sliced lengthwise
- Coarse salt and ground pepper
- ½ cup dry white wine
- 1 artichoke heart, rinsed and cut lengthwise
- 1 pint grape or cherry tomatoes, halved lengthwise, divided
- ⅓ cup pitted Kalamata olives, cut lengthwise
- ½ cup fresh basil leaves, torn
- ¼ cup grated Parmesan cheese, plus more for serving

Directions

- Cook pasta in a large pot of boiling salted water following package instructions, until al dente; drain and reserve 1 cup of pasta water.
- Return the cooked pasta to the pot.

- In the meantime, heat 1 tablespoon of extra virgin olive oil; add garlic and onion, season with sea salt and black pepper and cook, stirring regularly, for about 4 minutes.
- Stir in wine and continue cooking for about 2 minutes more or until the liquid is evaporated.
- Stir in the artichoke and continue cooking for about 3 minutes more or until starting to brown.
- Stir in half of the tomatoes, and olives and cook for 2 minutes.
- Add pasta and stir in the remaining olive oil, tomatoes, basil and cheese; Add the reserved pasta water, as desired, to coat the pasta.
- Serve immediately with extra cheese.

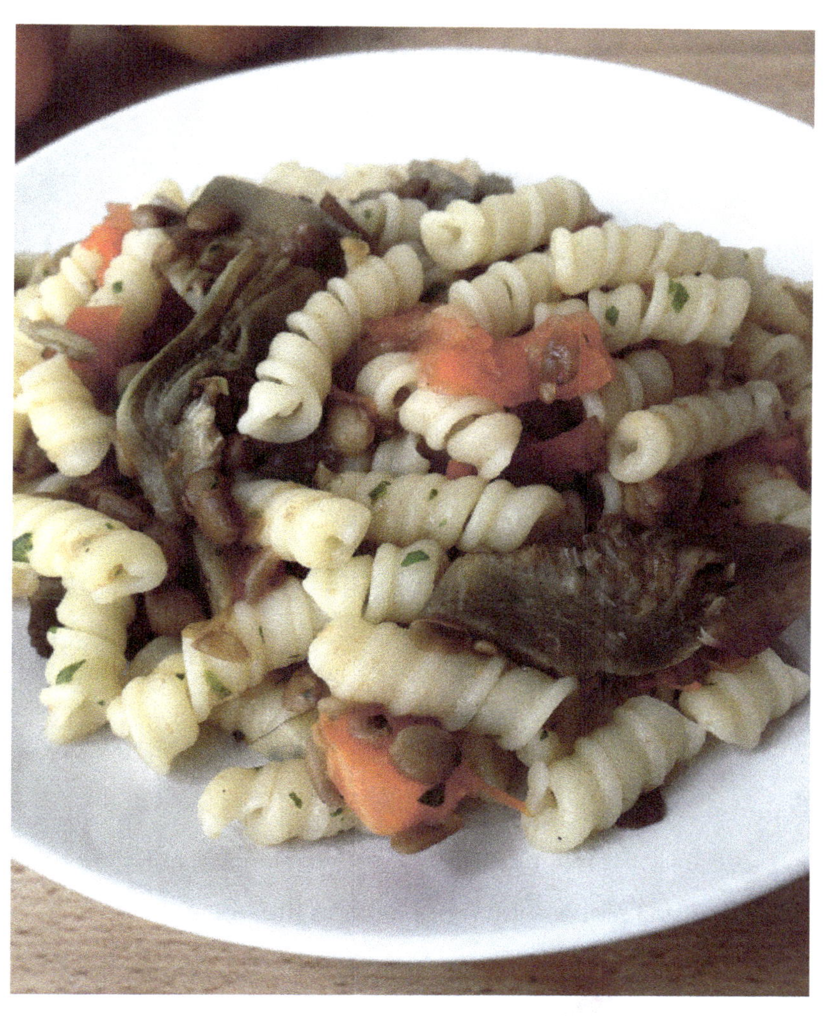

Swiss Chard with Olives

Total time: 30 minutes

Prep time: 15 minutes

Cook time: 15 minutes

Yield: 4 servings

Ingredients

- 1 ¼ pounds trimmed and rinsed Swiss chard
- 1 tsp. extra virgin olive oil
- 2 garlic cloves, sliced
- 1 small yellow onion, sliced
- 1 jalapeno pepper, chopped
- ⅓ cup Kalamata olives (brine-cured), pitted and roughly chopped
- ½ cup water

Directions

- Separate stems from leaves of Swiss chard; cut the stems into small pieces and roughly chop the leaves; set aside.
- Heat extra virgin olive oil to a Dutch oven or a large skillet over medium heat.
- Add garlic, onion, and jalapeno; sauté for about 6 minutes or until onion is tender and translucent.
- Add olives, Swiss chard stems, and water and cook, covered, for about 3 minutes.
- Stir in the chard leaves and continue cooking, covered, for about 4 minutes or until the leaves and stems are tender.
- Serve immediately.

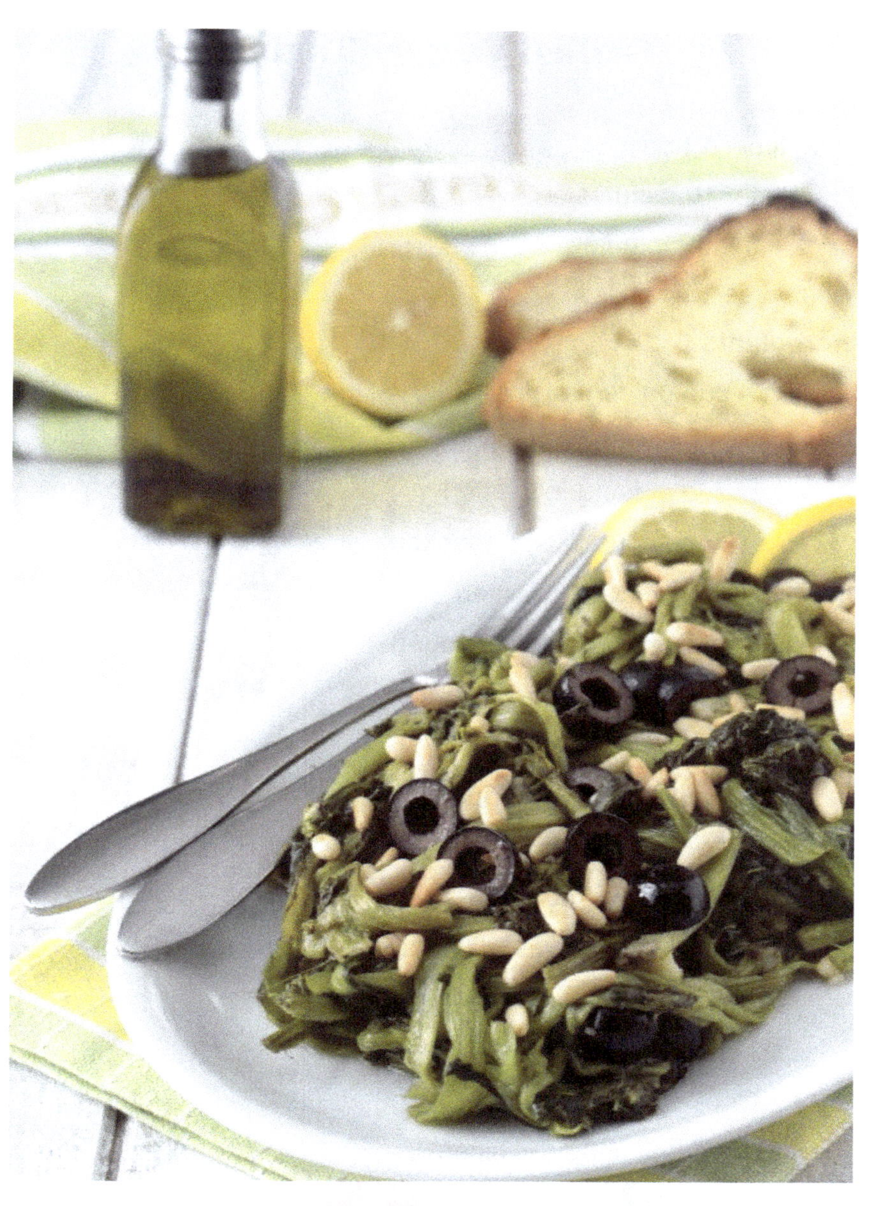

Grilled Veggies Tagine

Total time: 1 hour

Prep time: 10 minutes

Cook time: 50 minutes

Yield: 6 servings

Ingredients

- ¼ cup golden raisins
- 6 small red potatoes, cut in quarters
- ¼ cup pine nuts, toasted
- 2/3 cup couscous, uncooked
- 2 garlic cloves, pressed
- I medium red onion, wedged
- 1 tsp. fennel seeds, crushed
- ¼ tsp. cinnamon, ground
- 1 ¾ cups onions, chopped
- 1 tsp. extra virgin olive oil
- 1 tsp. cumin, ground
- ¼ cup green olives, pitted and chopped
- 1 ½ cups water
- ¼ tsp. freshly ground black pepper
- Cooking spray
- 2 red bell peppers, diced
- 1 green bell pepper, diced
- ½ tsp. kosher salt
- 2 tsp. balsamic vinegar
- ½ can tomatoes, chopped

Directions

- Prepare a gas or charcoal grill.
- Combine the bell peppers, red onion, and ¼ teaspoon sea salt, vinegar and ½ teaspoon olive oil in a zip lock plastic bag and toss well.
- Place a large nonstick saucepan on medium heat and add the remaining olive oil and add the garlic and chopped onion.
- Sauté these for about 3 minutes and add fennel, cumin and cinnamon.
- Let them cook for a further 1 minute then add the remaining salt, olives, raisins, potatoes, tomatoes, black pepper and water and bring the pan to a boil.
- Cover the saucepan, and simmer for 25 minutes or until the potatoes are tender
- Remove the onions and bell peppers from the plastic bag and grill on a rack coated with cooking spray for about 10 minutes.
- Boil the remaining water in a separate saucepan and slowly stir in the couscous.
- Remove from heat and cover the pan and let it stand for 5 minutes.
- Serve the tomato mixture over couscous and top with the grilled onions, bell peppers and pine nuts.

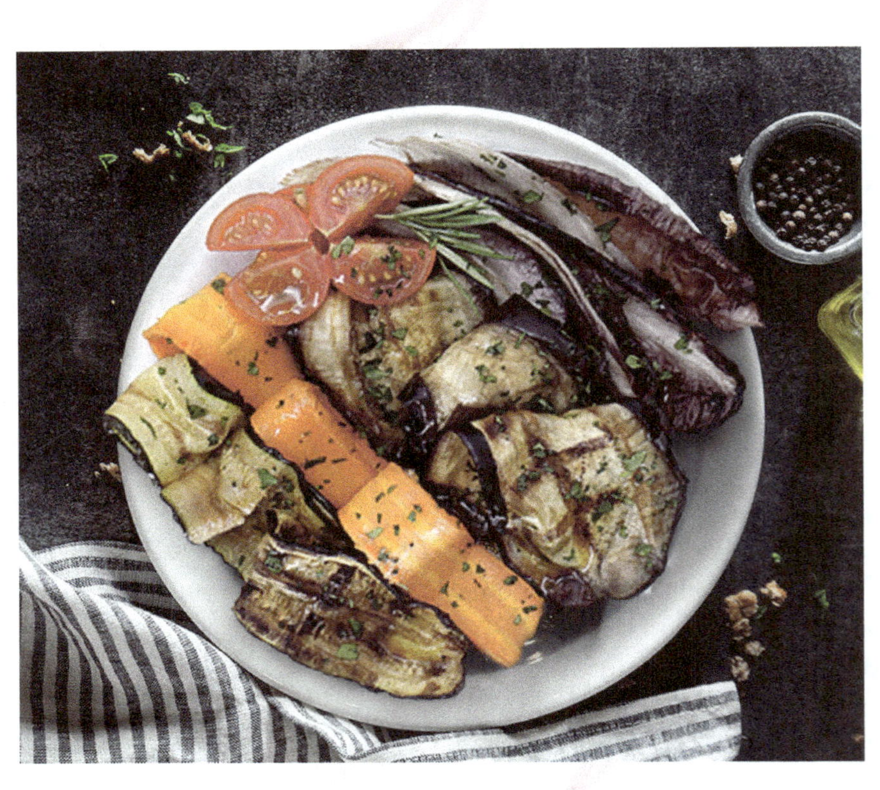

MEDITERRANEAN DESSERTS

Spinach Cake

Total time: 1 hour

Prep time: 15 minutes

Cook time: 45 minutes

Yields: 12 Spinach Cakes

Ingredients

- 1 ½ pounds spinach, rinsed
- 3 tbsp. extra virgin olive oil
- 1 cup pine nuts
- 2 cloves garlic, minced
- ½ cup currants
- 1 tsp. sea salt
- 2 large eggs, whisked

Directions

- Wilt spinach in a pan set over low heat for about 5 minutes; drain and let cool a bit before squeezing moisture out of the spinach.
- Pulse the spinach in a food processor until coarsely chopped; set aside.
- Warm oil in a skillet; add pine nuts and sauté for a few minutes or until golden brown.
- Stir in garlic and continue cooking for 1 more minute.
- Combine the pine nut mixture, currants, blended spinach, eggs and salt in a bowl; spread the mixture into a coated baking dish and bake at 350°F for about 35 minutes.

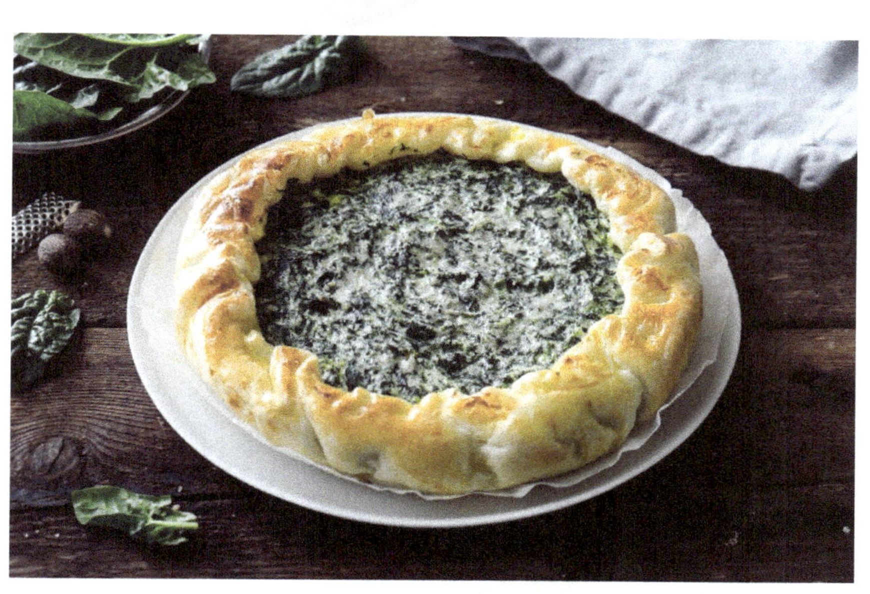

Citrus Tarts

Total time: 40 minutes

Prep time: 15 minutes

Cook time: 25 minutes

Yield: 6 servings

Ingredients

- 1 ½ packs frozen mini phyllo pastry shells
- 1 cup whipping cream, divided
- ½ tsp. almond extract, divided
- ¼ cup orange curd
- ¼ cup strawberry curd
- Fresh mint leaves for garnish

Directions

- Bake the pastry shells according to the package's instructions and set aside until they cool off completely.
- In a food processor, beat ½ cup whipping cream, ¼ teaspoon almond extract and orange curd until soft peaks start to form.
- Spoon this mixture into half the baked pastry shells.
- Again beat the remaining whipping cream, almond extract and strawberry curd in the food processor until soft peaks form and spoon in the remaining shells.
- Garnish with mint leaves and serve.

Pistachio and Fruits

Total time: 12 minutes

Prep time: 5 minutes

Cook time: 7 minutes

Yield: 12 servings

Ingredients

- 1 ¼ cups unsalted pistachios, roasted
- ½ cup apricots, dried and chopped
- ¼ cup dried cranberries
- ½ tsp. cinnamon
- 2 tsp. sugar
- ¼ tsp. allspice
- ¼ tsp. ground nutmeg

Directions

- Preheat your oven to 350°F and bake pistachios in a baking tray for about 6 minutes.
- Set aside and let them cool completely.
- Mix all the ingredients in a bowl until well combined and you are ready to serve.

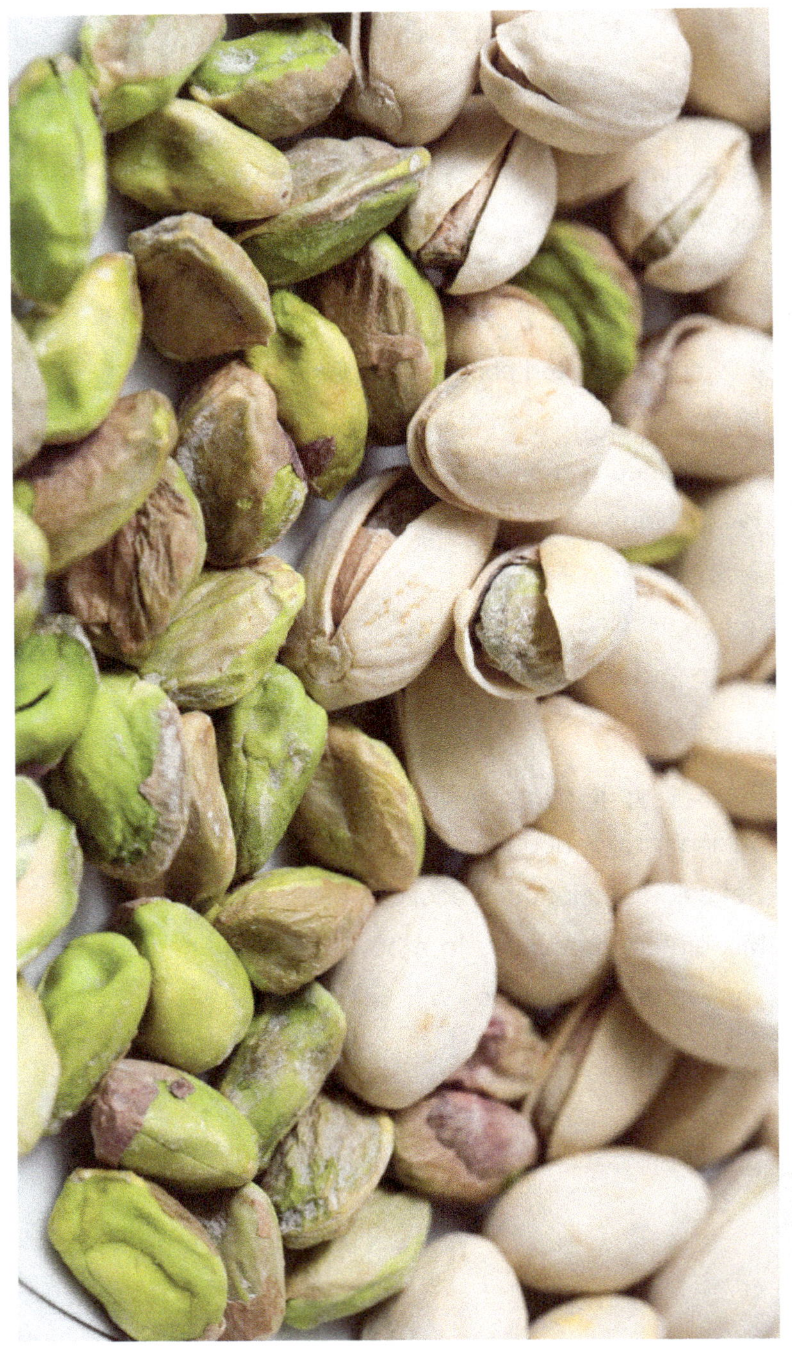

GREEK MESS

Serves 10

- 2 cups whipping cream
- 1 cup confectioners' sugar, divided
- 1 teaspoon ground mastiha
- 2 pints raspberries or other seasonal berry, divided
- 12 Greek almond cookies, crumbled, divided
- 1⁄2 cup chopped almonds
- 4 tablespoons chopped mint leaves

Directions

- In a medium bowl, beat the whipping cream until soft peaks form. Add 1⁄2 cup of sugar and the mastiha. Continuing whipping the mixture until stiff peaks form. Keep the mixture cool.

- In another medium bowl, combine 2⁄3 of the berries and the remaining sugar. Stir until the sugar is melted. Coarsely mash the berries into the consistency of a chunky jam.

- Gently fold the berry mixture into the whipped cream. Fold half of the crumbled cookies into the berry–whipped cream mixture.

- Divide the mixture into individual serving bowls or glasses, and top with the remaining crumbled cookies, remaining berries, almonds, and mint.

- Serve immediately or cover and refrigerate for up to 1 day.

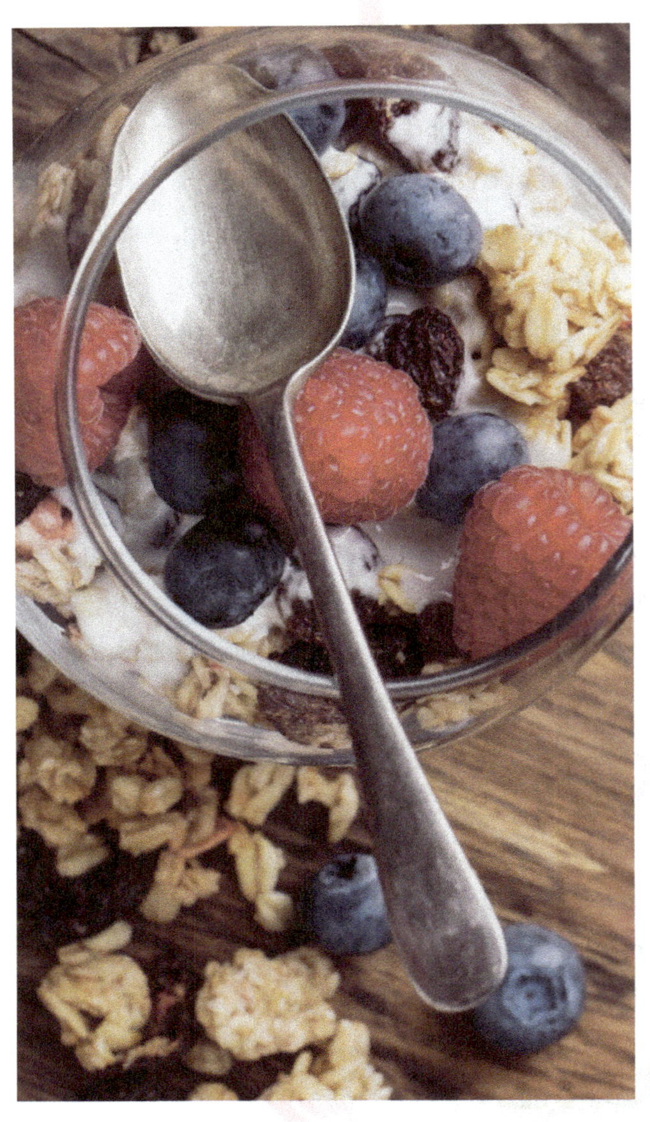

MEDITERRANEAN BREAD

PIZZA DOUGH

Makes 1 large or 2 medium pizzas

- 1½ teaspoons active dry yeast
- ½ teaspoon sugar
- 1½ cups warm water
- ½ teaspoon salt
- 3 tablespoons extra-virgin olive oil, divided
- 3¾ cups all-purpose flour, divided

Directions

- In a large bowl, add the yeast, sugar, and warm water. Set the mixture aside for 7–10 minutes to allow the yeast to activate (bubble or froth). Stir in the salt and 2 tablespoons of oil.
- Place ¼ cup of flour on your work surface. Add the remaining 3½ cups of flour, a little at a time, to the yeast mixture; mix the ingredients with your hands. When the mixture comes together as a dough, empty the bowl onto the floured work surface and begin to knead it. Keep kneading until the dough is pliable and no longer sticks to your hands. For a large pizza, roll the dough into one ball. For two medium pizzas, divide the dough in half and roll the halves into balls.
- To use the dough immediately, place each ball in a bowl and rub the surface of the dough with the remaining oil. Cover the bowl with plastic wrap, and let the dough rise in a warm place until it doubles in size (1½– 2 hours).

- The dough can be frozen to use later. Rub the surface of the dough with the remaining oil and wrap it in plastic. Place the wrapped dough into a plastic bag and freeze it until needed. Then thaw the dough and let it rise before using it.

LADENIA

Serves 12

- ½ cup extra-virgin olive oil, divided
- ¼ cup semolina flour Pizza Dough
- 2 large onions, peeled and thinly sliced
- 2 large tomatoes, cut in half and then cut into half-moon slices
- 1 teaspoon salt
- ½ teaspoon pepper
- 2 tablespoons dry oregano

Directions

- Cover the surface of a large baking pan evenly with ¼ cup of oil. Sprinkle the semolina flour evenly over the oil. Roll out the dough to the dimensions of the baking pan and transfer it to the pan, stretching it to fit.
- Cover the baking pan with a tea towel and allow the dough to rise for 30 minutes in a warm place. Preheat the oven to 400°F.
- Pour the remaining oil over the dough and spread it out evenly. Sprinkle the top with the onions followed by the tomatoes. Sprinkle with salt, pepper, and oregano.
- Bake the ladenia on the middle rack for 40–50 minutes or until the edges have browned and the top is lightly golden.
- Serve hot or at room temperature.

MEDITERRANEAN RICE AND GRAINS

Quinoa Salad with Watermelon and Feta

Serves: 4

Ingredients

- 1 cup Simple Truth Organic™ Quinoa
- 3 tablespoons apple cider vinegar
- 2 tablespoons lemon juice
- ½ Vidalia onion, finely chopped
- ½ cup Simple Truth Organic™ Unfiltered Extra Virgin Olive Oil
- Coarse salt, to taste
- Freshly ground pepper, to taste
- ¾ cup crumbled feta cheese
- ½ seedless watermelon, (about 1½ cups) diced
- 3 tablespoons Italian parsley, minced

Directions

Step 1

- Cook quinoa according to package directions. Rinse with cold water and drain.

Step 2

- To make dressing: in a small bowl or jar, combine vinegar, lemon juice and onion. Mix well and add in olive oil and whisk well to emulsify dressing. Season with salt and pepper to taste.

Step 3

- In a medium bowl, combine the cooked quinoa with feta, watermelon, parsley and dressing. Add salt and pepper to taste. Serve chilled or at room temperature.

MEDITERRANEAN EGGS RECIPES

Mediterranean Feta & Quinoa Egg Muffins

INGREDIENTS

- 2 cups baby spinach, finely chopped
- 1/2 cup finely chopped onion*
- 1 cup chopped or sliced tomatoes {cherry or grape tomatoes work well}
- 1/2 cup chopped {pitted} kalamata olives
- 1 tablespoon chopped fresh oregano
- 2 teaspoons high oleic sunflower oil, plus optional extra for greasing muffin tins
- 8 eggs
- 1 cup cooked quinoa*
- 1 cup crumbled feta cheese
- 1/4 teaspoon salt

INSTRUCTIONS

- Pre-heat oven to 350 degrees fahrenheit, and prepare 12 silicone muffin holders on a baking sheet, or grease a 12 cup muffin tin with oil and set aside.
- Chop vegetables and heat a skillet to medium. Add vegetable oil and onions and saute for 2 minutes. Add tomatoes and saute for another minute, then add spinach and saute until wilted, about 1 minute. Turn off heat and stir in olives and oregano, and set aside.
- Place eggs in a blender or mixing bowl and blend/mix until well combined. Pour eggs in to a mixing bowl {if using a

blender} then add quinoa, feta cheese, veggie mixture, and salt, and stir until well combined.

- Pour mixture in to silicone cups or greased muffin tins, dividing equally, and bake in oven for 30 minutes, or until eggs have set and muffins are a light golden brown. Allow to cool for 5 minutes before serving, or may be chilled and eaten cold, or re-heated in a microwave the next day.

MEDITERRANEAN BREAKFAST BAKE

Ingredients

- 2 tablespoons olive oil, divided
- 1 pound Italian turkey sausage or chicken sausage, removed from casings
- 1 small onion, chopped
- 1/2 teaspoon salt
- 1 5-ounce package baby spinach
- 8 eggs
- 1 cup milk
- 6 slices whole grain bread, cut into 1/2-inch pieces
- 1 cup chopped sundried tomato
- 1 14-ounce can quartered artichoke hearts, drained
- 1/2 cup crumbled feta cheese

Instructions

- Heat 1 tablespoon olive oil in large nonstick skillet over medium-high heat. Add sausage and cook, stirring and breaking up , until browned, about 8 minutes. Remove and set aside.
- Add remaining tablespoon olive oil to skillet and add onion and salt cook until softened, about 5 minutes. Add spinach and cook until just wilted, about 1 minute.
- Beat eggs and stir in milk. Stir in bread, sundried tomatoes, artichokes, feta cheese, sausage and spinach mixture.
- Pour mixture into a 2-1/2-quart baking dish coated with cooking spray, spreading egg mixture evenly in baking dish. Cover and refrigerate 1 hour or overnight.

- Preheat oven to 350°. Remove casserole from refrigerator; let stand 30 minutes. Bake at 350° for 45 minutes or until set and lightly browned. Let stand 10 minutes before serving.

Mediterranean-Brunch-Bake

Ingredients

- 2 500g Burnbrae Farms Egg Creations Whole Eggs Veggie & Feta
- 1 tbsp extra virgin olive oil
- 1 small red onion, chopped
- 2 zucchini, chopped
- 1 red pepper, chopped
- 2 tomatoes, seeded and diced
- 1 green pepper, chopped
- 1 tsp fresh thyme
- 1 tbsp fresh basil, chopped
- 1/2 cup black olives, sliced
- 1 cup feta cheese, crumbled
- 1/2 tsp salt
- 1/4 tsp pepper

Instructions

- Preheat oven to 375F. Spray a 9 x 13 casserole dish with cooking spray.
- Heat olive oil over medium high heat in a skillet. Add red onion, zucchini, red pepper and green pepper. Sauté until softened, about 5 to 7 minutes. Spread in the greased casserole dish.
- Pour both cartons of Egg Creations on top. Spread thyme, basil, tomatoes, black olives, feta cheese, salt and pepper over top.

Mediterranean-frittata

Ingredients

- 12wholeeggs
- 1jarroasted red peppers12 oz size, drained
- 6ouncesgoat cheesecrumbled
- 1/4cupfreshly grated parmesan cheese
- 1pinchsalt
- olive oilas needed for coating the pan
- 4ouncescremini mushroomssliced
- 1/4pounddeli hamdiced

Instructions

- Pre-heat the oven to 350 F. In a large mixing bowl combine the eggs, roasted red peppers, goat cheese, parmesan and salt. Whisk that all together thoroughly.

- Get out a cast iron skillet (8 or 10 inches would both work) and coat it liberally in olive oil, including brushing it all over the sides. Heat the pan over medium high heat and add the mushrooms. Let them get soft for a minute, then add the diced ham and let it fry up for another minute.

- Pour the egg mixture into the hot pan and make sure everything is well mixed and even. Then carefully transfer the pan to the oven and let the frittata bake for 30-35 minutes, until golden and puffy.

- Take the frittata out when it's done and let it set for a few minutes. Then just cut it into wedges right in the pan and serve immediately! Enjoy the eggy, Mediterranean goodness.

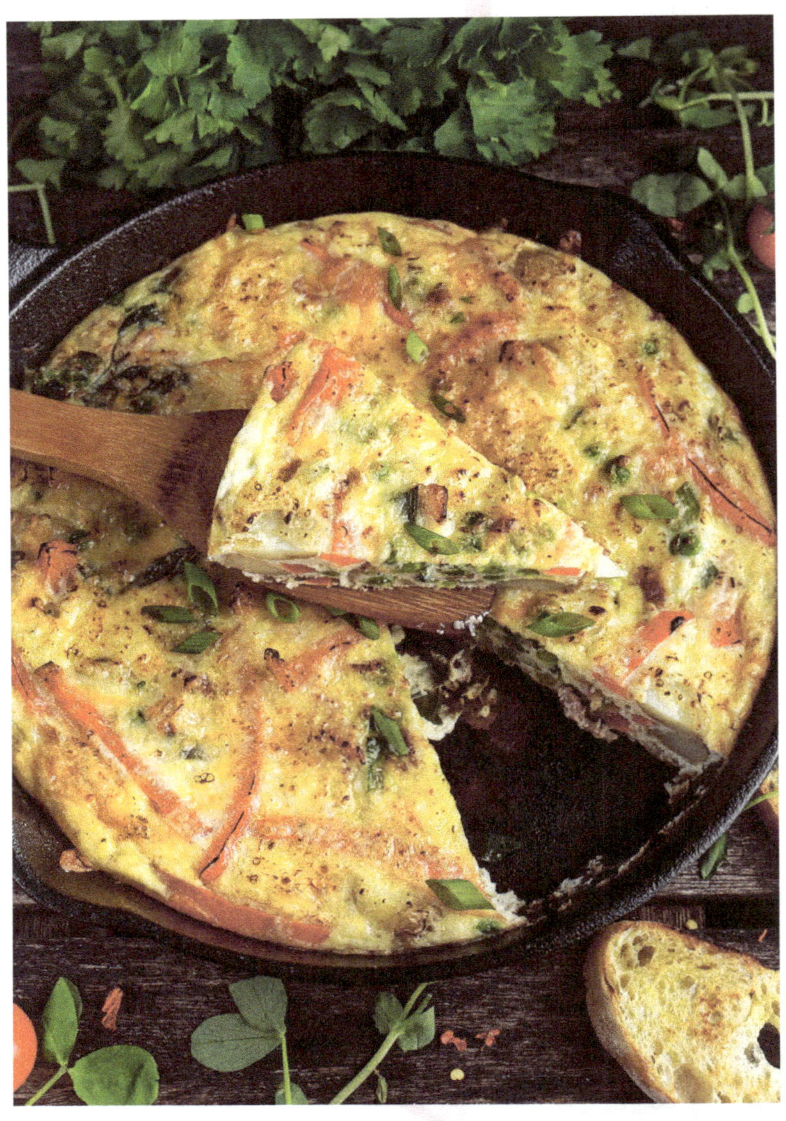

Mediterranean Strata

Ingredients

- 3 tablespoons butter
- 2 cloves garlic minced
- 2 shallots minced
- 1 cup button mushrooms sliced
- 1 teaspoon dried marjoram leaves
- 6 cups white bread cut into 1/2 inch chunks
- 1/2 cup artichoke hearts cut into 1/8ths
- 1/4 cup kalamata olives quartered
- 1/4 cup marinated sun dried tomatoes slivered
- 1/4 cup shredded Parmesan cheese plus additional for topping
- 4 ounces or 1 cup Ciliegine Fresh Mozzarella cheese balls halved
- 6 eggs
- 1 1/2 cups half and half
- 1/4 cup basil leaves slivered
- Kosher salt

Instructions

- Melt 1 tablespoon butter. For individual stratas, brush insides of four 1-cup baking dishes. If serving family style, brush inside of 2-quart baking dish.
- Preheat oven to 325°F.
- In large skillet over medium heat, melt remaining 2 tablespoons butter. Add garlic and shallot; sauté for 2

minutes. Add mushrooms and marjoram and cook for another 4 minutes. Remove from heat and place mushroom mixture in large bowl with bread chunks, artichoke hearts, kalamata olives, sun dried tomatoes, Parmesan and Fresh Mozzarella and stir to mix. Season lightly with kosher salt. Fill baking dishes evenly with the bread mixture.

* In 4-cup liquid measuring cup, mix eggs with half and half and pour 1 cup of egg mixture evenly over bread in each dish. Garnish with basil and more Parmesan.

* Place baking dishes on a baking sheet and bake for 50 minutes or until eggs have set. Remove from oven and let rest 5 minutes before serving.

MEDITERRANEAN APPETIZERS

Feta and Greek Yogurt Dip

Total time: 10 minutes

Prep time: 10 minutes

Cook time: 0 minutes

Yields: 8 servings

Ingredients

- ¼ cup crumbled tomato-basil feta cheese
- 2 tbsp. reduced-fat mayonnaise
- 1 (6-oz) container Greek fat-free plain yogurt
- 2 tbsp. fresh parsley, chopped
- Assorted fresh vegetables

Directions

- Mix together cheese, mayonnaise, yogurt and parsley in a small bowl until well blended.
- Divide the dip among bowls and serve with your favorite vegetables.

Eggplant and Olive Dip

Total time: 40 minutes

Prep time: 15 minutes

Cook time: 25 minutes

Yield: Approximately 2 Cups

Ingredients

- 2 (10 ounces each) Italian eggplants, cut into halves lengthwise
- 1 ½ tsp. extra virgin olive oil, divided
- ½ cup pitted green olives, such as Sicilian or Picholine
- ½ cup pitted Kalamata olives
- Pinch of red-pepper flakes
- 1 tsp. finely grated lemon zest
- 1 garlic clove, thinly sliced
- 1/4 tsp. coarse salt
- 1 tsp. fresh oregano, finely chopped
- Small oregano leaves for garnish
- Long zest strips for garnish
- 2 yellow bell peppers, ribs and seeds removed, diced

Directions

- Preheat your oven to 400°F.
- Arrange the eggplants, cut-side down, on a baking sheet and brush with ½ teaspoon of extra virgin olive oil.
- Spread garlic on top and season with sea salt; roast in the preheated oven for about 20 minutes or until tender and golden.

- Remove from heat and let cool for at least 5 minutes.

- Remove and discard the eggplant seeds and spoon the flesh into a food processor, along with garlic; pulse until smooth and transfer to a bowl.

- Add the olives to the processor and process until roughly chopped; add to the eggplant mixture and stir in the remaining extra virgin olive oil, red pepper flakes, lemon zest, and the chopped oregano.

- Garnish with lemon zest strips and fresh oregano leaves and serve with bell peppers.